The Complete KETO Sweet Chaffle Cookbook

Easy And Mouth-watering Sweet Chaffle Recipes For Beginners

Lily Sherman

1

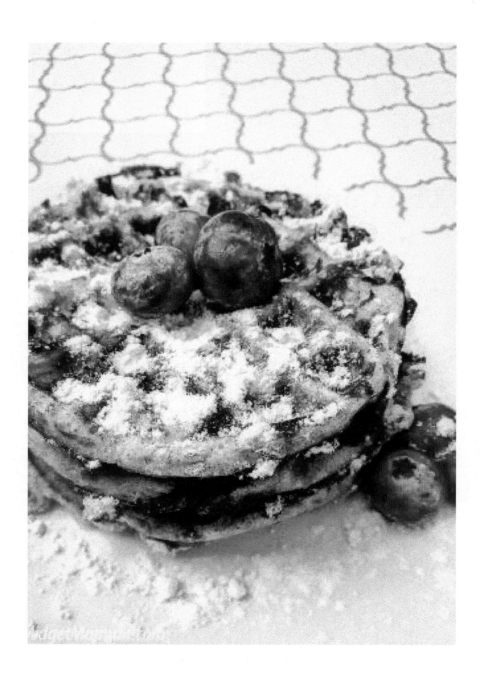

Table of contents

Mouth-Watering Strawberry Chaffle

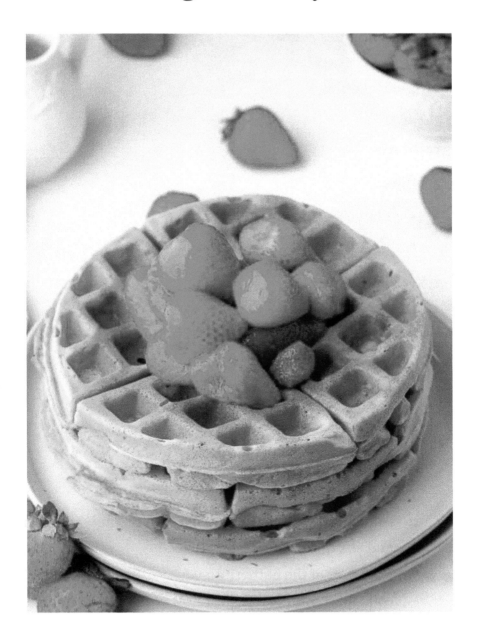

Preparation: 5 minutes

Cooking: 8 minutes

Servings: 2 chaffles

Ingredients

For chaffles:

- 1 large egg, beaten
- ½ cup of mozzarella cheese, shredded
- 2 tbsp almond flour
- ¼ tsp baking powder

For topping:

- 2 tbsp almond butter
- 2 tbsp fresh strawberries, sliced

Directions

1. Heat up your waffle maker.
2. Add all the chaffles ingredients to a tiny mixing bowl and stir until well combined.
3. Pour half of the batter into your waffle maker and cook for 4 minutes. Repeat now with the rest of the batter to make another chaffle.

4. Let cool for 3 minutes to let chaffles get crispy.
5. Spread the chaffle with almond butter and garnish with fresh strawberries.
6. Serve and enjoy!

Crunchy Peach Chaffle

Preparation: 5 minutes

Cooking: 8 minutes

Servings: 2 chaffles

Ingredients

<u>For chaffles:</u>

- 1 tbsp almond flour
- ½ cup mozzarella cheese
- 1 egg, beaten
- ½ teaspn vanilla extract

<u>For topping:</u>

- 1 ripe peach, sliced
- 1 tbsp unsweetened peach syrup
- ½ tbsp almond, minced

Directions

1. Heat up your waffle maker.
2. Add all the chaffles ingredients to a tiny mixing bowl and combine well.

3. Pour ½ of the batter into your waffle maker and cook for 4 minutes until brown. Then cook the remaining batter to make another chaffle.
4. Top the chaffle with peach slices, a tbsp of unsweetened peach syrup and sprinkle with minced almonds.
5. Serve and enjoy!

Orange Glaze Chaffle

Preparation: 5 minutes

Cooking: 8 minutes

Servings: 2 chaffles

Ingredients

For chaffles:

- 1 tbsp almond flour
- ½ cup mozzarella cheese
- 1 egg, beaten
- ½ tsp vanilla extract

For glaze:

- 1tbsp unsalted butter, softened
- 1 tbsp sweetener
- 2 tbsp cream cheese, softened
- ¼ tsp orange extract

Directions

For glaze:

1. Add all the ingredients in a blender and whisk until creamy.

For chaffles:

1. Heat up your waffle maker.
2. Add all the chaffles ingredients to a tiny mixing bowl and combine well.
3. Pour ½ of the batter into your waffle maker and cook for 4 minutes until brown. Then cook the remaining batter to make another chaffle.
4. Top the chaffle with orange frosting.
5. Serve and enjoy!

Chocolate Chaffle with Orange Glaze

Preparation: 5 minutes

Cooking: 8 minutes

Servings: 2 chaffles

Ingredients

For chaffles:

- 1 egg, beaten
- ½ cup of mozzarella cheese, shredded
- 2 tbsp chocolate chips, unsweetened
- 1 tbsp sweetener
- 1 tbsp whipping cream
- 1 tbsp almond flour
- ½ tsp vanilla extract
- ¼ tsp baking powder

For glaze:

- 1tbsp unsalted butter, softened
- 1 tbsp sweetener
- 2 tbsp cream cheese, softened
- ¼ tsp orange extract

Directions

<u>For glaze:</u>

1. Add all the ingredients to a blender and whisk until creamy.

<u>For Chaffle:</u>

1. Heat up your waffle maker.
2. Add all the chaffles ingredients to a tiny mixing bowl and mix well.
3. Pour half of the batter into your waffle maker and cook for 4 minutes until golden brown. Repeat now with the rest of the batter to make another chaffle.
4. Let cool for 3 minutes to let chaffles get crispy.
5. Spread the chaffles with orange frosting.
6. Serve and enjoy!

Buttercream Frosting Chaffle

Preparation: 5 minutes

Cooking: 8 minutes

Servings: 2 chaffles

Ingredients

For chaffles:

- 1 tbsp almond flour
- ½ cup mozzarella cheese
- 1 egg, beaten
- 1 tbsp sweetener
- ½ tsp vanilla extract

For frosting:

- 2 tbsp butter, softened
- 2 tbsp sweetener
- ¼ tsp vanilla extract

Directions

<u>For frosting:</u>

    1. Mix all the frosting ingredients until the mixture is creamy. Set aside.

<u>For chaffles:</u>

    1. Heat up your waffle maker.
    2. Add all the chaffles ingredients to a tiny mixing bowl and combine well.
    3. Pour ½ of the batter into your waffle maker and cook for 4 minutes. Then cook the remaining batter to make another chaffle.
    4. Top the chaffles with buttercream frosting.
    5. Serve and enjoy!

Nutmeg & Cinnamon Chaffle

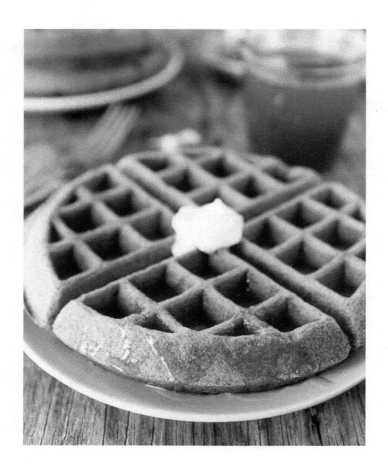

Preparation: 5 minutes

Cooking: 8 minutes

Servings: 2 chaffles

Ingredients

- 1 tbsp almond flour
- ½ cup mozzarella cheese, shredded
- 1 large egg, beaten
- ¼ tsp baking powder
- ¼ tsp nutmeg powder
- ½ tsp cinnamon powder

Directions

1. Heat up your waffle maker.
2. Add all the chaffles ingredients to a tiny mixing bowl and combine well.
3. Pour ½ of the batter into your waffle maker and cook for 4 minutes until golden brown. Then cook the remaining batter to make another chaffle.
4. Serve with maple syrup and enjoy!

Strawberry Mousse Chaffle

Preparation: 5 minutes

Cooking: 8 minutes

Servings: 2 chaffles

Ingredients

For chaffles:

- 1 large egg, beaten
- ½ cup mozzarella cheese, grated
- 1 tsp coconut flour
- 1 tsp water
- ¼ tsp baking powder

For mousse:

- 2 tbsp heavy whipping cream
- 2-3 tbsp fresh strawberries
- ½ tsp lemon zest
- ½ tsp vanilla extract
- 1-2 fresh mint leaves, for garnish

Directions

<u>For mousse:</u>

1. In a bowl, whip all the mousse ingredients until fluffy. Set aside.

<u>For chaffles:</u>

2. Heat up the mini waffle maker.
3. Add all the chaffles ingredients to a tiny mixing bowl and combine well.
4. Pour half of the batter into your waffle maker and cook for 4 minutes until brown. Repeat now with the rest of the batter to make another chaffle.
5. Let cool for 3 minutes to let chaffles get crispy.
6. Top the chaffles with strawberry mousse and garnish with a fresh mint leaf.
7. Serve and enjoy!

Raspberry Butter Chaffle

Preparation: 5 minutes

Cooking: 8 minutes

Servings: 2 chaffles

Ingredients

For chaffles:

- 1 large egg, beaten
- ½ cup mozzarella cheese, shredded
- 1 tsp coconut flour
- 1 tsp water
- ¼ tsp baking powder

For raspberry butter:

- 3 tbsp butter, softened
- 1 tbsp fresh raspberries

Directions

For raspberry butter:

1. In a tiny mixing bowl, combine all the ingredients. Mix with an electric mixer and set aside.

22

For chaffles:

2. Heat up your waffle maker.
3. Add all the chaffles ingredients to a tiny mixing bowl and combine well.
4. Pour half of the batter into your waffle maker and cook for 4 minutes until brown. Repeat now with the rest of the batter to make another chaffle.
5. Let cool for 3 minutes to let chaffles get crispy.
6. Spread the chaffles with raspberry butter.
7. Serve and enjoy!

Blueberry Butter Chaffle

Preparation: 5 minutes

Cooking: 8 minutes

Servings: 2 chaffles

Ingredients

Ingredients for chaffles:

- 1 large egg, beaten
- ½ cup mozzarella cheese, shredded
- 1 tsp coconut flour
- 1 tsp water
- ¼ tsp baking powder

Ingredients for blueberry butter:

- 3 tbsp butter, softened
- 1 tbsp fresh blueberries

Directions

Directions for blueberry butter:

1. In a tiny mixing bowl, combine all the ingredients. Mix with an electric mixer and set aside.

For chaffles:

1. Heat up your waffle maker.
2. Add all the chaffles ingredients to a tiny mixing bowl and combine well.
3. Pour half of the batter into your waffle maker and cook for 4 minutes until brown. Repeat now with the rest of the batter to make another chaffle.
4. Let cool for 3 minutes to let chaffles get crispy.
5. Spread the chaffles with blueberry butter.
6. Serve and enjoy!

Lemon Chaffle with Icing

Preparation: 9 minutes

Cooking: 4 minutes

Servings: 1 chaffle

Ingredients

- 1 egg
- ½ cup mozzarella cheese, shredded
- 1 tbsp cream cheese
- 2 tbsp almond flour
- 1 tbsp lemon juice
- 2 tsp sweetener
- ½ tsp lemon zest
- ¼ tsp baking powder
- A pinch of salt

For lemon icing:

- 2 tbsp powdered erythritol
- 4 tsp heavy cream
- 1 tsp lemon juice
- Lemon zest

Directions

1. Heat up your waffle maker.
2. Mix egg, cream cheese, mozzarella cheese, almond flour, lemon juice, sweetener, lemon zest, baking powder and salt in a tiny mixing bowl and blend until creamy.
3. Pour the batter into your waffle maker and cook for about 4 minutes.
4. Combine in a mixing bowl the powdered erythritol, heavy cream, lemon juice and lemon zest. Pour over lemon chaffle.
5. Serve and enjoy!

Chocolate Chaffle

Preparation: 5 minutes

Cooking: 16 minutes

Servings: 4 chaffles

Ingredients
- 2 eggs
- 1 cup butter
- ½ cup sugar-free chocolate chips
- ¼ cup sweetener
- 1 tsp vanilla extract

Directions
1. Heat up your waffle maker.
2. Place butter and chocolate chips on a plate and Melt now them in microwave for approx. 1 minute. Combine well.
3. In a tiny mixing bowl, beat egg.
4. Add beaten egg, vanilla, sweetener and chocolate mixture in a tiny mixing bowl and combine well.

28

5. Pour ¼ of the batter onto the bottom plate of your waffle maker.
6. Cook for approx. 4 minutes or until the chaffle is golden brown.
7. Repeat now with the rest of the batter.
8. Serve with your favorite berries and enjoy!

Chaffle Roll with Cinnamon

Preparation: 5 minutes

Cooking: 8 minutes

Servings: 2 chaffles

Ingredients

For the chaffles:

- ½ cup mozzarella cheese
- 2 tbsp almond flour
- ¼ tsp baking powder
- 1 egg
- 1 tsp cinnamon
- 1 tsp sweetener

For the glaze:

- 1 tbsp butter
- 1 tbsp cream cheese
- ¼ tsp vanilla extract
- 2 tsp sweetener

Directions

1. Heat up your waffle maker.
2. Add all the chaffle ingredients to a tiny mixing bowl and stir until well combined.
3. Pour half of the batter into your waffle maker and cook for 4 minutes until golden brown. Repeat now with the rest of the batter to make another chaffle.
4. Let cool for 3 minutes to let chaffle get crispy.
5. In the meantime, mix 1 tbspn butter and 1 tbspn of cream cheese in a tiny bowl. Heat in the microwave for 10-15 seconds until soft enough.
6. Add the vanilla extract and the sweetener to the butter and cream cheese and mix well using a whisk.
7. Drizzle keto cream cheese glaze on top of chaffle. Roll it.
8. Serve and enjoy!

Blackberry Roll Chaffle

Preparation: 5 minutes

Cooking: 16 minutes

Servings: 4 chaffles

Ingredients

For the chaffles:

- 1 egg
- 1 egg yolk
- 3 tbsp Melted butter
- 1 tbsp swerve confectioner's sugar substitute
- 1 cup parmesan cheese, grated
- 2 tbsp mozzarella cheese, shredded

For the cream:

- ½ cup ricotta cheese
- 2 tbsp swerve confectioner's sugar substitute
- 1 tsp vanilla extract
- 2 tbsp fresh blackberries, chopped

Directions

For the cream:

1. In a tiny mixing bowl stir ricotta cheese, vanilla extract and swerve confectioner's sugar substitute until creamy.
2. Add the blackberries and mix well.

For chaffles:

3. Heat up your waffle maker.
4. Add all the chaffle ingredients to a tiny mixing bowl and stir until well combined.
5. Pour 1/4 of the batter into your waffle maker and cook for 4 minutes until brown. Repeat now with the rest of the batter to make the other chaffles.
6. Let cool for 3 minutes to let chaffle get crispy.
7. Spread some filling on each chaffle and wrap over.
8. Serve and enjoy!

Lemon Icing Chaffle Roll

Preparation: 5 minutes

Cooking: 8 minutes

Servings: 2 chaffles

Ingredients

For chaffles:

- 1 large egg, beaten
- 2 tbsp cream cheese, softened
- 2 tbsp almond flour
- 2 tsp sweetener
- ¼ tsp baking powder

For lemon icing:

- 2 tbsp sweetener
- 4 tsp heavy cream
- 1 tsp lemon juice
- Fresh lemon zest

Directions

1. Heat up your waffle maker.

2. Add all the chaffles ingredients to a tiny mixing bowl and stir until well combined.
3. Pour half of the batter into your waffle maker and cook for about 4 min, until golden brown.
4. Repeat now with the rest of the batter to prepare another chaffle.
5. Combine in a mixing bowl the sweetener, heavy cream, lemon juice and lemon zest. Pour over the chaffles and roll them.
6. Serve and enjoy!

Cherry Chocolate Chaffle Roll

Preparation: 5 minutes

Cooking: 8 minutes

Servings: 2 chaffles

Ingredients

For chaffles:

- ½ cup shredded mozzarella cheese
- 1 tbsp almond flour
- 1 egg, beaten
- ¼ tsp cinnamon
- ½ tbsp sweetener
- 1 tbsp low carb chocolate chips
- 1 tbsp dark sweet cherries, halved

For roll:

- 2 tbsp whipped heavy cream, unsweetened
- 2 tsp sweetener

Directions

1. Heat up your waffle maker.

36

2. Add all the ingredients to a tiny mixing bowl and stir until well combined.

3. Add half of the batter into your waffle maker and cook it for approx. 4-5 minutes. When the first one is completely done cooking, cook the second one.

4. Set aside for 1-2 minutes.

5. Spread the chaffles with whipped heavy cream and sprinkle with sweetener. Roll them.

6. Serve and enjoy!

Ricotta & Berries Chaffle Roll

Preparation: 5 minutes

Cooking: 8 minutes

Servings: 2 chaffles

Ingredients

- 1 large egg, beaten
- ½ cup skim ricotta cheese
- 1 tbsp almond flour
- ½ tsp baking powder
- 1 tbsp fresh blackberries, chopped
- 1 tbsp fresh raspberries, chopped
- 2 tbsp sweetener for topping

Directions

1. Heat up your waffle maker.
2. Add all the ingredients to a tiny mixing bowl and stir until well combined.

3. Pour half of the batter into your waffle maker and cook for 4 minutes until golden brown. Repeat now with the rest of the batter to make another chaffle.
4. Let cool for 3 minutes to let chaffle get crispy.
5. Sprinkle the chaffle with sweetener and roll it.
6. Serve with keto maple syrup and enjoy!

Peanut Butter Chaffle Roll

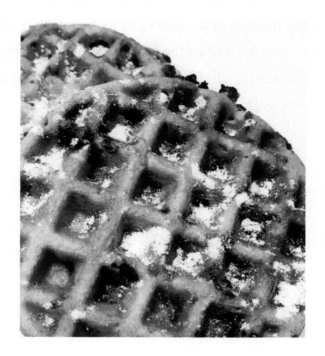

Preparation: 5 minutes

Cooking: 8 minutes

Servings: 2 chaffles

Ingredients

- 1 large egg, beaten
- ½ cup shredded mozzarella cheese

- 2 tbsp almond flour
- ½ tsp baking powder
- 1 tbsp cream cheese, softened
- 2 tbsp keto peanut butter for topping

Directions

1. Heat up your waffle maker.
2. Add all the chaffle ingredients to a tiny mixing bowl and stir until well combined.
3. Pour half of the batter into your waffle maker and cook for 4 minutes until golden brown. Repeat now with the rest of the batter to make another chaffle.
4. Spread the chaffle with peanut butter and roll it.
5. Serve and enjoy!

Buttercream Chaffle Roll

Preparation: 5 minutes

Cooking: 8 minutes

Servings: 2 chaffles

Ingredients

<u>For chaffles:</u>

- 1 tbsp almond flour
- ½ cup mozzarella cheese
- 1 egg, beaten
- 1 tbsp sweetener
- ½ tsp vanilla extract

<u>For frosting:</u>

- 2 tbsp butter, softened
- 2 tbsp sweetener
- ¼ tsp vanilla extract

<u>For roll:</u>

- 2 tbsp fresh raspberries, minced
- 2 tsp cocoa powder, unsweetened

Directions

For frosting:

1. Mix all the frosting ingredients until the mixture is creamy. Set aside.

For chaffles:

1. Heat up your waffle maker.
2. Add all the chaffle ingredients to a tiny mixing bowl and combine well.
3. Pour ½ of the batter into your waffle maker and cook for 4 minutes. Then cook the remaining batter to make another chaffle.
4. Top the chaffle with buttercream frosting. Add raspberries, sprinkle with cocoa powder and roll it.
5. Serve and enjoy!

Apple Cinnamon Chaffles

Preparation: 6 minutes

Cooking: 20 Minutes

Servings: 2

Ingredients

- 3 eggs, lightly beaten
- 1 cup mozzarella cheese, shredded
- ¼ cup apple, chopped
- ½ tsp monk fruit sweetener
- 1 ½ tsp cinnamon
- ¼ tsp baking powder, gluten-free
- 2 tbsp coconut flour

Directions

- Preheat now your waffle maker.
- Add remaining Ingredients and stir until well combined.
- Spray waffle maker with cooking spray.
- Pour 1/3 of batter in the hot waffle maker and cook for minutes or until golden brown. Repeat now with the remaining batter.

- Serve and enjoy.

Nutrition:

Calories 227, Fat 18.6, Fiber 4.5, Carbs 9.5, Protein 9.9

Banana Nut Chaffles

Preparation: 5 minutes

Cooking: 10 Minutes

Servings: 1

Ingredients

- 1 egg
- 1 Tbsp. cream cheese, softened and room temp
- 1 Tbsp. sugar-free cheesecake pudding
- ½ cup Mozzarella cheese
- 1 Tbsp. monk fruit confectioners' sweetener
- ¼ tsp. vanilla extract
- ¼ tsp. banana extract
- toppings of choice

Directions

1. Turn on waffle maker to heat and oil it with cooking spray.
2. Beat egg in a tiny bowl.
3. Add remaining ingredients and Mix well until well incorporated.

4. Add one half of the batter to waffle maker and cooking for min, until golden brown.
5. Remove now chaffle and add the other half of the batter.
6. Top with your optional toppings and serve warm!

Nutrition:

Calories: 246, Total fat: 23g, Protein: 7g, Total carbs: 8g

Custard Chaffle Roll

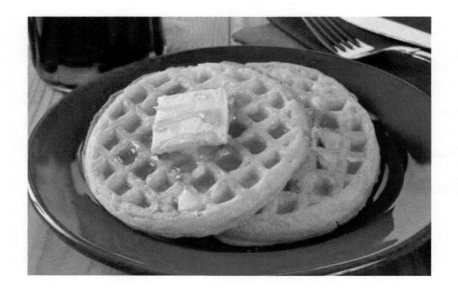

Preparation: 5 minutes

Cooking: 55 minutes

Servings: 2 chaffles

Ingredients

For chaffles:

- 2 tbsp almond flour
- ½ cup mozzarella cheese
- 1 egg, beaten

- 1 tbsp sweetener
- ½ tsp vanilla extract

For custard:

- 2 eggs
- 2 tbsp heavy cream
- 1 tbsp brown sugar substitute
- ½ tsp cinnamon powder
- ½ tsp vanilla extract

For topping:

- 2 tsp of coconut flour

Directions

For custard:

1. Preheat now the oven at 350°.
2. Place all ingredients in a tiny bowl and stir until well combined.
3. Pour the mixture in a baking tin and bake it for about 40-45 minutes.
4. Remove now from heat and set aside to cool.

For chaffles:

5. Heat up your waffle maker.
6. Add all the chaffle ingredients to a tiny mixing bowl and combine well.

49

7. Pour ½ of the batter into your waffle maker and cook for 4 minutes until golden brown. Then cook the remaining batter to make another chaffle.
8. Top the chaffles with custard and sprinkle with coconut flour. Roll them.
9. Serve and enjoy!

Mint Chaffles Cake

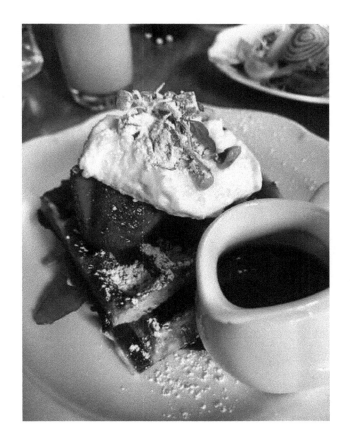

Preparation: 5 minutes

Cooking: 16 minutes

Servings: 4 chaffles

Ingredients

<u>For chaffles:</u>

- 2 tbsp almond flour
- 1 cup mozzarella cheese, shredded
- 2 eggs, beaten
- 2 tbsp sweetener
- 1 tsp vanilla extract
- 8 chopped mint leaves
- A pinch of salt

<u>For filling:</u>

- 3 fresh chopped strawberries
- ½ tbsp sweetener
- 2 tbsp keto whipped cream

Directions

<u>For filling:</u>

1. Place the strawberries in a bowl and add ½ tbspn of sweetener. Mix and set aside.

<u>For chaffles:</u>

2. Heat up your waffle maker.
3. Add all the ingredients to a tiny mixing bowl and combine well.

4. Pour ¼ of the batter into your waffle maker and cook for 4 minutes until golden brown. Then cook the remaining batter to prepare the other chaffles.
5. Assemble the cake by placing whipped cream and strawberries on top of your mint chaffles. Then drizzle the juice that will also be in the bowl with the strawberries on top.
6. Serve and enjoy!

Caramel Chaffles Cake

Preparation: 4 minutes

Cooking: 16 minutes

Servings: 4 chaffles

Ingredients

For chaffles:

- 2 eggs, beaten
- 1 cup mozzarella cheese, grated
- 2 tsp coconut flour
- 2 tsp water
- ½ tsp baking powder

For filling:

- 4 tbsp keto caramel sauce
- 4 tbsp coconut whipped cream
- 1 tsp coconut flakes

Directions

1. Heat up your waffle maker.

2. Add all the chaffles ingredients to a tiny mixing bowl and combine well.
3. Pour 1/4 of the batter into your waffle maker and cook for 4 minutes until brown. Repeat now with the rest of the batter to prepare the other chaffles.
4. Let cool for 3 minutes to let chaffles get crispy.
5. Top the chaffle with caramel sauce and whipped cream. Cover with another chaffle and repeat the procedure.
6. Serve with coconut flakes and enjoy!

Pumpkin Chaffles Cake

Preparation: 5 minutes

Cooking: 8 minutes

Servings: 2 chaffles

Ingredients

For chaffles:

- 1 egg, beaten
- ½ cup mozzarella cheese, shredded
- 1 tbsp almond flour
- ½ tsp baking powder
- ¼ cup pumpkin puree
- 1 tbsp heavy cream
- 1 tsp cream cheese
- ½ tsp vanilla extract

For filling cake:

- 2 tbsp cream cheese, softened
- 1 tbsp sweetener
- ½ tsp vanilla extract
- 1 tsp keto maple syrup

Directions

For cake filling:

1. Whisk all the ingredients until creamy.

For chaffles:

2. Heat up your waffle maker.
3. Add all the chaffles ingredients to a tiny mixing bowl and stir until well combined.
4. Pour half of the batter into your waffle maker and cook for 4 minutes until golden brown. Repeat now with the rest of the batter to make another chaffle.
5. Let cool for 3 minutes to let chaffles get crispy.
6. Spread the chaffle with cream and cover with another chaffle. Sprinkle with sweetener or cocoa powder.
7. Serve and enjoy!

Strawberry Chaffles Cake with Frosting

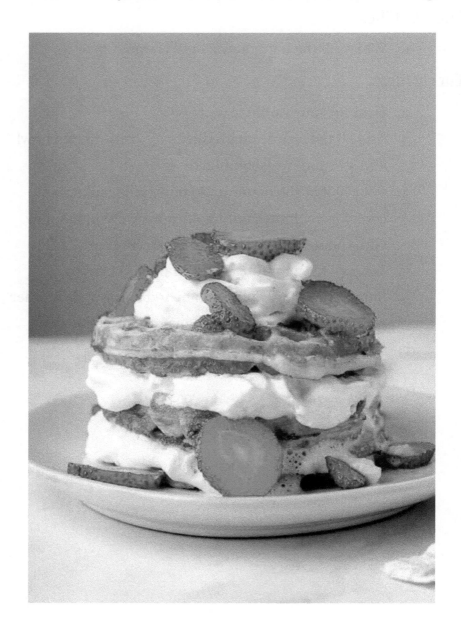

Preparation: 5 minutes

Cooking: 12 minutes

Servings: 3 chaffles

Ingredients

For chaffles:

- ½ cup mozzarella cheese
- 1 egg, beaten
- 1 tbsp cream cheese
- ¼ tsp baking powder
- 2 fresh strawberries, sliced
- 1 tsp strawberry extract

For frosting:

- ¼ tbsp strawberry extract
- 1 tbsp cream cheese
- 1 tbsp sweetener

For the whipped cream:

- 1 tsp vanilla
- 1 tbsp sweetener
- 1 cup heavy whipping cream

Directions

1. Heat up your waffle maker.
2. Add all the ingredients to a tiny mixing bowl and combine well.
3. Pour 1/3 of the batter into your waffle maker and cook for 4 minutes until golden brown. Then cook the remaining batter to make the other chaffles.
4. In a tiny mixing bowl whisk the ingredients for the whipped cream until fluffy.
5. Prepare the frosting by mixing the whipping cream with vanilla and the sweetener.
6. Assemble the cake by placing whipped cream and strawberries on top of your sweet chaffle. Then drizzle the juice that will also be in the bowl with the strawberries on top.
7. Serve and enjoy!

Chocolatey Chaffle

Preparation: 5 min

Cooking: 4 min

Servings: 2

Ingredients

- 1 large egg
- 1 oz. cream cheese, softened
- 1 tbsp ChocZero Chocolate Syrup
- 1/2 tsp vanilla
- 1 tbsp Stevia sweetener
- 1/2 tbsp cacao powder
- 1/4 tsp baking powder

Directions

- Preheat now mini waffle maker until hot
- Whisk egg in a bowl, add cheese, then mix well
- Stir in the remaining ingredients (except toppings, if any).

- Scoop 1/2 of the batter onto your waffle maker, spread across evenly
- Cook until a bit browned and crispy, about 4 minutes.
- Gently Remove now from waffle maker and let it cool
- Repeat now with remaining batter.
- Serve and Enjoy!

Nutrition:

241 Calories, 2g Net Carbs, 19g Fat, 13g Protein

Chocolate Chip Cannoli Chaffles

Preparation: 15 minutes

Cooking: 5 minutes

Servings: 4

Ingredients

For the chocolate chip chaffle:

- 1 tbsp butter, Melted
- 1 tbsp monkfruit
- 1 egg yolk
- 1/8 tsp vanilla extract
- 3 tbsp almond flour
- 1/8 tsp baking powder
- 1 tbsp chocolate chips, sugar-free

For the cannoli topping:

- 2 oz cream cheese
- 2 tbsp low-carb confectioners sweetener
- 6 tbsp ricotta cheese, full fat
- 1/4 tsp vanilla extract
- 5 drops lemon extract

Directions

1. Preheat now the mini waffle maker.
2. Mix all the ingredients for the chocolate chip chaffle in a mixing bowl. Combine well to make a batter.
3. Place half the batter on your waffle maker. Allow to cook for 3-4 minutes.
4. While waiting for the chaffles to cook, start making your cannoli topping by combining all ingredients until the consistency is creamy and smooth.
5. Place the cannoli topping on the cooked chaffles before serving.

Nutrition:

Calories: 187, Carbohydrates: 7g, Fat: 13g , Protein: 7g

Lemon Chaffle Dome Cake

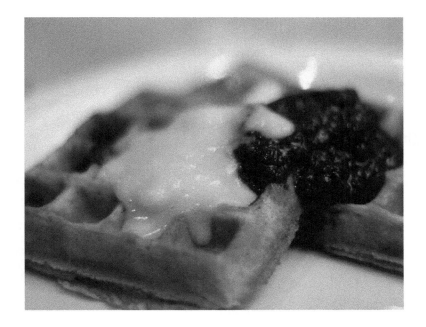

Preparation: 30 minutes

Cooking: 30 minutes

Servings: 4

Ingredients

For the chaffles:

- 2 eggs
- 2 oz cream cheese, softened

- 1 tbsp coconut flour
- 2 tsp heavy cream
- 2 tsp lemon juice
- 1/2 tsp vanilla extract
- 1/4 tsp stevia powder
- 1/4 tsp baking soda

For the lemon frosting:

- 8 oz cream cheese, softened
- 2 oz unsalted butter, softened
- 1 tbsp stevia powder
- 1 tbsp lemon zest
- 1 tsp lemon juice
- 1/2 tsp vanilla extract

Directions

1. Preheat now the mini waffle maker.
2. Combine all the chaffle ingredients using a blender.
3. Onto the Preheat nowed waffle maker, pour 1/4 of the batter.
4. Close the lid. Let the batter cook for 4-5 minutes. Remove now the cooked chaffle using a pair of silicone tongs.
5. Repeat the steps to use up the remaining batter.

6. Let the chaffles cool completely.

7. Make the lemon frosting by combining the ingredients in a bowl.

8. Assemble by cutting two of the chaffles in half.

9. Use cling wrap to line a tiny bowl.

10. Place a whole chaffle in the bowl, carefully molding it to the bowl's shape.

11. Line each side with the four chaffle halves.

12. Add half the amount of lemon frosting.

13. Cover the frosting with the last whole chaffle.

14. Cover the bowl with cling wrap. Put in the fridge for 30 minutes. You don't need to chill the remaining lemon frosting.

15. Invert the chaffle dome onto a plate.

16. Spread the remaining lemon frosting over it. Add decorations if desired.

17. Chill the cake for another 30 minutes. Serve.

Blackberries and Chaffles

Preparation: 5 minutes

Cooking: 8 Minutes

Servings: 2

Ingredients

- 1 organic egg, beaten
- 1/3 cup of Mozzarella cheese, shredded
- 1 teaspn cream cheese, softened
- 1 teaspn coconut flour
- ¼ teaspn organic baking powder
- ¾ teaspn powdered Erythritol
- ¼ teaspn ground cinnamon
- ¼ teaspn organic vanilla extract
- Pinch of salt
- 1 tbspn fresh blackberries

Directions

1. Preheat now a mini waffle iron and then grease it.
2. Place all ingredients except for blackberries and beat until well combined in a bowl.

3. Fold in the blackberries.
4. Place half of the mixture into Preheated waffle iron and cooking for about minutes or until golden brown.
5. Repeat now with the remaining mixture.
6. Serve warm.

Nutrition:

Calories: 418, Fat: 30.7g, Carbohydrates: 2.7g

Pumpkin Cream Chaffles

Preparation: 5 minutes

Cooking: 10 Minutes

Servings: 2

Ingredients

- 1 organic egg, beaten
- ½ cup Mozzarella cheese, shredded
- 1½ tbspn sugar-free pumpkin puree
- 2 teaspns heavy cream
- 1 teaspn cream cheese, softened
- 1 tbspn almond flour
- 1 tbspn Erythritol
- ½ teaspn pumpkin pie spice
- ½ teaspn organic baking powder
- 1 teaspn organic vanilla extract

Directions

1. Preheat now a mini waffle iron and then grease it.

2. In a bowl, place all ingredients and with a fork, Mix well until well combined.
3. Place half of the mixture into Preheated waffle iron and cooking for about 5 minutes or until golden brown.
4. Repeat now with the remaining mixture.
5. Serve warm.

Nutrition:

Calories: 286, Fat: 12.7g, Carbohydrates: 16.8g

Vanilla Chaffle

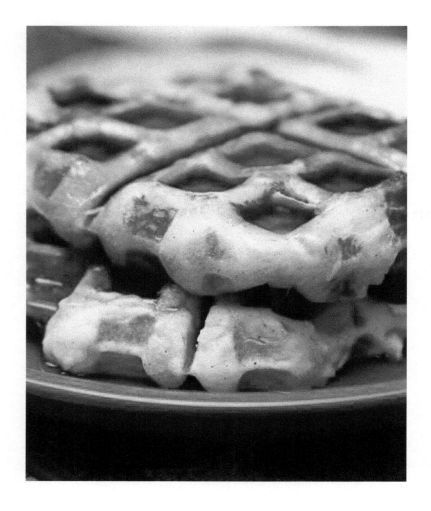

Cooking: 8 Minutes

Servings: 2

Ingredients

- 2 tbsp butter, softened
- 2 oz cream cheese, softened
- 2 eggs
- ¼ cup almond flour
- 2 tbsp coconut flour
- 1 tsp baking powder
- 1 tsp vanilla extract
- ¼ cup confectioners
- Pinch of pink salt

Directions

1. Preheat now your waffle maker and spray with non-stick cooking spray.
2. Melt now the butter and set aside for a minute to cool.
3. Add the eggs into the melted butter and whisk until creamy.
4. Pour in the sweetener, vanilla, extract, and salt. Blend properly.
5. Next add the coconut flour, almond flour, and baking powder. Mix well.
6. Pour into your waffle maker and cook for 4 minutes.
7. Repeat the process with the remaining batter.

8. Remove now and set aside to cool.

9. Enjoy.

Nutrition:

Calories: 202 Kcal, Fats: 27 g, Carbs: 9 g, Protein: 23 g

Cinnamon Pecan Chaffle

Preparation: 5 minutes

Cooking: 40 Minutes

Servings: 1

Ingredients

- 1 Tbsp. butter
- 1 egg
- ½ tsp. vanilla
- 2 Tbsp. almond flour
- 1 Tbsp. coconut flour
- ⅛ tsp. baking powder
- 1 Tbsp. monk fruit
- For the crumble:
- ½ tsp. cinnamon
- 1 Tbsp. Melted butter
- 1 tsp. monk fruit
- 1 Tbsp. chopped pecans

Directions

1. Turn on waffle maker to heat and oil it with cooking spray.
2. Melt now butter in a bowl, then mix in the egg and vanilla.
3. Mix in remaining chaffle ingredients.
4. Combine crumble ingredients in a separate bowl.
5. Pour half of the chaffle mix into waffle maker. Top with half of crumble mixture.
6. Cooking for 5 min, or until done.
7. Repeat now with the other half of the batter.

Nutrition:

Calories: 353, Fat: 10g, Carbohydrates: 4g

Chaffle-Glazed with Raspberry

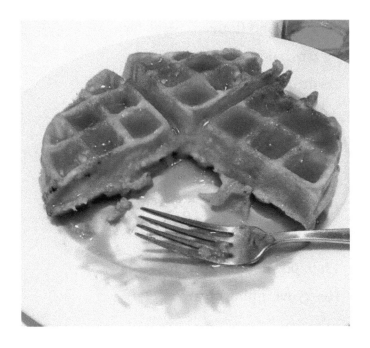

Preparation: 5 minutes

Cooking: 5 Minutes

Servings: 1

Ingredients

Donut Chaffle:

- 1 egg
- ¼ cup Mozzarella cheese, shredded

- 2 tsp. cream cheese, softened
- 1 tsp. sweetener
- 1tsp. almond flour
- ½ tsp. baking powder
- 20 drops glazed donut flavoring

Raspberry Jelly Filling:

- ¼ cup raspberries
- 1 tsp. chia seeds
- 1 tsp. confectioners' sweetener

Donut Glaze:

- 1 tsp. powdered sweetener
- Heavy whipping cream

Directions

1. Spray your waffle maker with cooking oil and add the butter mixture into your waffle maker.
2. Cooking for 3 minutes and set aside.

Raspberry Jelly Filling:

3. Mix all the ingredients for it
4. Place in a pot and heat on medium.
5. Gently mash the raspberries and set aside to cool.

Donut Glaze:

6. Stir together the ingredients

<u>Assembling:</u>

7. Lay your chaffles on a plate and add the fillings mixture between the layers.
8. Drizzle the glaze on top and enjoy.

Nutrition:

Calories: 350, Fat: 17.6g, Carbohydrates: 18.1g

Sage Plus Coconut Milk Chaffles

Cooking: 24 Minutes

Servings: 6

Ingredients

- ¾ cup coconut flour, sifted
- 1½ teaspns organic baking powder
- ½ teaspn dried ground sage
- 1/8 teaspn garlic powder
- 1/8 teaspn salt
- 1 organic egg
- 1 cup unsweetened coconut milk
- ¼ cup water
- 1½ tbsps coconut oil, Melted
- ½ cup cheddar cheese, shredded

Directions

1. Preheat now a waffle iron and then grease it.
2. In a bowl, add the flour, baking powder, sage, garlic powder, salt, and mix well.
3. Add the egg, coconut milk, water and coconut oil and Mix well until a stiff mixture form.

4. Add the cheese and gently stir to combine.

5. Divide the mixture into 6 portions.

6. Place 1 portion of the mixture into Preheated waffle iron and cook for about 4 minutes or until golden brown.

7. Repeat now with the remaining mixture.

8. Serve warm.

Nutrition:

Calories 126, Fat 5.1g, Fiber 1.6g, Carbs 5.9g, Protein 4.4 g

Pumpkin-Pecan Chaffle

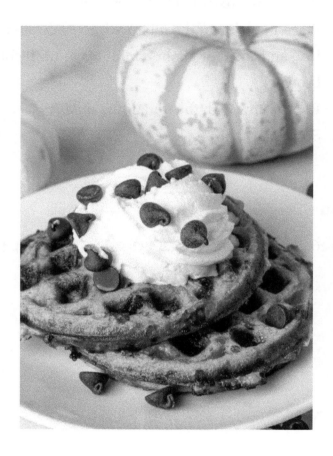

Preparation: 6 minutes

Cooking: 10 Minutes

Servings: 2

Ingredients

- 2 tbsp. toasted pecans (chopped)
- 2 tbsp. almond flour
- 1 tbsp. pumpkin puree
- ½ tsp. pumpkin spice
- ½ cup grated Mozzarella cheese
- 1 tsp. granulated swerve sweetener
- 1 egg
- ½ tsp. nutmeg
- ½ tsp. vanilla extract
- ½ tsp. baking powder

Directions

1. Plug your waffle maker to preheat it and spray it with a non-stick spray.
2. In a mixing bowl, combine the almond flour, baking powder, pumpkin spice, swerve, cheese and nutmeg.
3. In another mixing bowl, whisk together the pumpkin puree egg and vanilla extract.
4. Pour the egg mixture into the flour mixture and Mix well until the ingredients are well combined.
5. Pour an appropriate amount of the batter into your waffle maker and spread out the batter to the edges to cover all the holes on your waffle maker.

6. Close your waffle maker and cooking for about 5 minutes or according to your waffle maker's settings.
7. After the cooking cycle, use a silicone or plastic utensil to remove now the chaffle from your waffle maker.
8. Repeat step 5 to 7 until you have cooked all the batter into chaffles.
9. Serve warm and top with whipped cream. Enjoy!!!

Nutrition:

Calories 85, Fat 6.7g, Fiber 0.7g, Carbs 2.6g, Protein 5.3g

Brownie Batter Chaffle

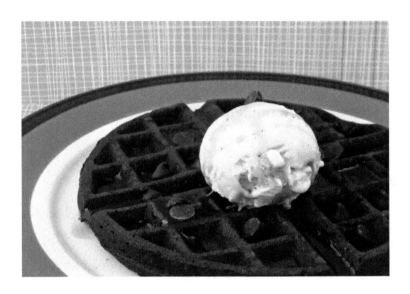

Preparation: 10 minutes

Cooking: 25 minutes

Servings: 16

Ingredients

- 1/2 cup / 50 grams almond flour
- ½ cup / 75 grams chopped chocolate, unsweetened
- 1 teaspn baking powder
- 1/4 teaspn salt

- 1/4 cup / 40 grams cocoa powder, unsweetened
- 1/4 teaspn liquid stevia
- 1/2 cup / 100 grams Swerve Sweetener
- 1/2 teaspn vanilla extract, unsweetened
- 12 tbsps coconut butter
- 5 eggs, at room temperature

Directions

1. Take a non-stick waffle iron, plug it in, select the medium or medium-high heat setting and let it Preheat now until ready to use; it could also be indicated with an indicator light changing its color.
2. Meanwhile, prepare the batter and for this, take a saucepan, place it over medium heat, add cocoa powder, chocolate, and butter and cook for 3 to 4 minutes until the butter has melted, whisking frequently.
3. Then add sweetener, stevia, and vanilla into the pan, stir until combined, remove now the pan from heat and let it stand for 5 minutes.
4. Take a bowl, add flour in it and then stir in baking powder and salt until mixed.
5. After 5 min, beat eggs into the chocolate-butter mixture and stir the flour until incorporated.

6. Use a spoon to pour ¼ cup of the prepared batter into the heated waffle iron in a spiral direction, starting from the edges, then shut the lid and cook for 5 minutes or more until solid and nicely browned; the cooked waffle will look like a cake.
7. When done, transfer chaffles to a plate with a silicone spatula and Repeat now with the remaining batter.
8. Let chaffles stand for some time until crispy and serve straight away.

Pumpkin Pie Chaffle

Preparation: 5 min

Cooking: 4 min

Servings: 2

Ingredients

- 1/2 cup Mozzarella cheese (shredded)
- 1 large Egg
- 2 1/2 tbsp Erythritol
- 1/2 oz Cream cheese
- 3 tsp Coconut flour
- 2 tbsp Pumpkin puree
- 1/4 tsp Baking powder (optional)
- 1/2 tbsp Pumpkin pie spice
- 1/2 tsp Vanilla extract (optional)
- 2 tbsp Heavy whipping cream (topping)
- Dash of cinnamon (topping)

Directions

1. Preheat now mini waffle maker until hot

2. Whisk egg in a bowl, add cheese, then mix well
3. Stir in the remaining ingredients (except toppings, if any).
4. Pour half of the batter onto your waffle maker, spread evenly
5. Cook until a bit browned and crispy, about 4 minutes.
6. Gently Remove now from waffle maker and let it cool
7. Repeat now with remaining batter.
8. Top with whipped cream and cinnamon

Nutrition:

117 Calories, 3g Net Carbs, 7g Fat, 7g Protein

Fudgy Chocolate Chaffles

Preparation: 5 mins

Cooking: 8 mins

Servings: 2

Ingredients

- 1 egg
- 2 tbsp mozzarella cheese, shredded
- 2 tbsp cocoa
- 2 tbsp Lakanto monk fruit powdered
- 1 tsp coconut flour
- 1 tsp heavy whipping cream
- 1/4 tsp baking powder
- 1/4 tsp vanilla extract
- pinch of salt

Directions

1. Turn on waffle or chaffle maker. I use the Dash Mini Waffle Maker. Grease lightly or use a cooking spray.
2. In a tiny bowl, combine all ingredients.

3. Cover the dash mini waffle maker with 1/2 of the batter. Close the mini waffle maker and cook for 4 minutes. Remove now the chaffle from your waffle maker carefully as it is very hot.

4. Repeat the steps above.

5. Serve with sugar-free strawberry ice cream or sugar-free whipped topping.

Light & Crispy Bagel Chaffle Chips

Preparation: 5 minutes

Cooking: 5 minutes

Servings: 4

Ingredients

- 3 tbsp. parmesan cheese
- 1 tsp. oil for grease
- 1 tsp. bagel seasoning
- Salt and pepper to taste

Directions

1. Preheat now your waffle maker.
2. Add the parmesan cheese in the pan and melt now it well.
3. Now pour the melted parmesan cheese over your waffle maker and sprinkle bagel seasoning over the cheese.
4. Cooking the mixture for about 2 to 3 minutes without closing the lid.

5. Let it settle or turn crispy for 2 minutes then Remove now and serve the crispy chis crunch.

Nutrition:

Net Carbs: 1.2 g; Calories: 201.2; Total Fat: 12.9g; Saturated Fat: 9.1g; Protein: 19.6g; Carbs: 1.5g; Fiber: 0.3g; Sugar: 0.7g

Lime Pie Chaffle Recipe

Preparation: 10 minutes

Cooking: 5 minutes

Servings: 2

Ingredients

Key Lime Pie Chaffle:

- 1 egg
- 1/4 cup Almond flour
- 2 tsp cream cheese room temp
- 1 tsp powdered sweetener swerve or monk fruit
- 1/2 tsp lime extract or 1 tsp fresh squeezed lime juice
- 1/2 tsp baking powder
- 1/2 tsp lime zest
- Pinch of salt to bring out the flavors

Cream Cheese Lime Frosting:

- 4 oz cream cheese softened
- 4 tbs butter
- 2 tsp powdered sweetener swerve or monk fruit
- 1 tsp lime extract

- 1/2 tsp lime zest

Directions

1. Preheat now the mini waffle iron.
2. In a blender, add all the chaffle ingredients and blend on high until the mixture is smooth and creamy.
3. Cook each chaffle about 3 to 4 minutes until it's golden brown.
4. While the chaffles are cooking, make the frosting.
5. In a tiny bowl, combine all the ingredients for the frosting and mix it until it's smooth.
6. Allow the chaffles to completely cool before frosting them.

Keto Vanilla Twinkie Copycat Chaffle Recipe

Preparation: 10 minutes

Cooking: 4 minutes

Servings: 4

Ingredients

- 2 tbsps butter Melted (cooled)
- 2 ounce ofs cream cheese softened
- 2 large eggs room temp
- 1 teaspn vanilla extract
- 1/2 teaspn Vanilla Cupcake Extract (optional)
- 1/4 cup Lakanto Confectioners
- Pinch of pink salt
- 1/4 cup almond flour
- 2 tbsps coconut flour
- 1 teaspn baking powder

Directions

1. Preheat now the Corndog Maker.

2. Melt now the butter and let it cool a minute.

3. Whisk the eggs into the butter until creamy.

4. Add vanilla, extract, sweetener, salt, and then blend well.

5. Add Almond flour, coconut flour, and baking powder.

6. Blend until well incorporated.

7. Add 2 tbsp batter to each well and spread across evenly.

8. Close lid, lock, and let cook 4 minutes.

9. Remove now and cool on a rack.

Peppermint Mocha Chaffles with Buttercream Frosting

Preparation: 10 minutes

Cooking: 10 minutes

Servings: 6

Ingredients

Chaffles:

- 1 egg
- 1 ounce of cream cheese at room temperature
- 1 tbspn Melted butter or coconut oil
- 1 tbspn unsweetened cocoa powder or raw cacao
- 2 tbsps powdered sweeteners such as Swerve or Lakanto
- 1 tbspn almond flour
- 2 teaspns coconut flour
- 1/4 teaspn baking powder powder
- 1 teaspn instant coffee granules
- 1/4 teaspn vanilla extract
- Pinch salt

Filling:

- 2 tbsps butter at room temperature
- 2-3 tbsps powdered sweeteners such as Swerve or Lakanto
- 1/4 teaspn vanilla extract
- 1/8 teaspn peppermint extract
- Optional toppings: sugar-free starlight mints

Directions

For the Mocha Chaffles:

1. Heat the waffle iron until thoroughly hot.
2. Beat all chaffle ingredients together in a tiny bowl until smooth.
3. Add a heaping 2 tbsps of batter to waffle iron and cook until done about 4 minutes.
4. Repeat to make 3 chaffles. Let cool on wire rack.

For the Buttercream Frosting:

5. In a tiny bowl with a hand mixer, beat the butter and sweetener until smooth.
6. Add the heavy cream and vanilla extract and beat at high speed for about 4 min, until light and fluffy.
7. Spread frosting on each chaffle and garnish with sugar-free starlight mints, if desired.

Raspberry-Pecan Chaffles

Preparation: 10 minutes

Cooking: 14 minutes

Servings: 2

Ingredients

- 1 egg, beaten
- ½ cup finely grated mozzarella cheese
- 1 tbsp cream cheese, softened
- 1 tbsp sugar-free maple syrup
- ¼ tsp raspberry extract
- ¼ tsp vanilla extract
- 2 tbsp sugar-free caramel sauce for topping
- 3 tbsp chopped pecans for topping

Directions

1. Preheat now the waffle iron.
2. In a bowl, mix all the ingredients.
3. Open the iron, pour in half of the batter, close, and cook until crispy, 6 to 7 minutes.
4. Remove now the chaffle onto a plate and set aside.

5. Make another chaffle with the remaining batter.
6. To serve: drizzle the caramel sauce on the chaffles and top with the pecans.

Cranberry Swirl Chaffles with Orange Cream Cheese Frosting

Preparation: 10 minutes

Cooking: 20 minutes

Servings: 6

Ingredients

Cranberry sauce:

- 1/2 cup cranberries fresh or frozen
- 2 Tbsp granulated erythritol
- 1/2 cup water
- 1/2 tsp vanilla extract

Chaffles:

- 1 egg
- 1 ounce of cream cheese at room temperature
- 1 Tbsp erythritol blends such as Swerve, Pyure or Lakanto
- 1/2 tsp vanilla extract
- 1 tsp coconut flour
- 1/4 tsp baking powder

Frosting:

- 1 ounce of cream cheese at room temperature
- 1 Tbsp butter room temperature
- 1 Tbsp confectioner's sweetener such as Swerve
- 1/8 tsp orange extract OR 2 drops orange essential oil
- A few strands of grated orange zest (optional)

Directions

For the cranberry swirl:

1. Combine the cranberries, water, and erythritol in a medium saucepan. Bring to a boil, then reduce heat to a gentle simmer.
2. Simmer for 10-15 min, until the cranberries pop and the sauce thickens.
3. Remove now from heat and stir in the vanilla extract.
4. Mash the berries with the back of a spoon until a chunky sauce forms.
5. The sauce will thicken off the heat significantly.

For the chaffles:

6. Preheat the waffle iron until thoroughly hot.
7. In a bowl, whisk all chaffle ingredients together until well combined.
8. Spoon 2 tbsps of batter into a waffle iron.

9. Add 1/2 of the cranberry sauce in little dollops over the batter of each chaffle.

10. Close and cook 3-5 min, until done. Remove now to a wire rack.

11. Repeat for the second chaffle.

For the Frosting:

12. Mix all ingredients, except orange zest, until smooth and spread over each chaffle.

13. Orange zest (optional).

Chocolate Cherry Chaffles

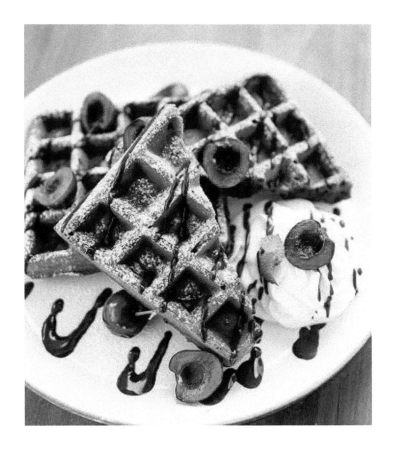

Preparation: 5 minutes

Cooking: 5 Minutes

Servings: 1

Ingredients

- 1 Tbsp almond flour

- 1 Tbsp cocoa powder

- 1 Tbsp sugar free sweetener

- ½ tsp baking powder

- 1 whole egg

- ½ cup mozzarella cheese shredded

- 2 Tbsp heavy whipping cream whipped

- 2 Tbsp sugar free cherry pie filling

- 1 Tbsp chocolate chips

Directions

1. Turn on waffle maker to heat and oil it with cooking spray.

2. Mix all dry components in a bowl.

3. Add egg and mix well.

4. Add cheese and stir again.

5. Spoon batter into waffle maker and close.

6. Cook for 5 min, until done.

7. Top with whipping cream, cherries, and chocolate chips.

Nutrition:

Calories: 307, Fat: 17g, Protein: 7g, Carbohydrates: 35g, Fiber: 11g

Lightning Source UK Ltd.
Milton Keynes UK
UKHW020813110621
385331UK00004B/77